NORTH SHORE
ASTHMA CLINIC
*Center for Evaluation,
Education and Treatment*

why do I wheeze?

A GUIDE TO THE EFFECTIVE MANAGEMENT OF ASTHMA

ROBERT SORENSEN, M.D.

WHY DO I WHEEZE?

Copyright © 2000
Robert H. Sorensen, M.D.
First Printing 2000

All Rights Reserved. No part of this book may be reproduced in any form without written permission from the author or publisher.

Published by: North Shore Asthma Clinic
1950 Sheridan Rd Suite 202
Highland Park, IL 60035
(847) 266-3580
www.whydoiwheeze.com

Cover Design: TORTORICI-LAPORTE DESIGN

ISBN: 0-9678835-0-4

Library of Congress Card Number: 00-190296

Printed in the United States by
Morris Publishing
3212 East Highway 30
Kearney, NE 68847
1-800-650-7888

Dedication

This book is dedicated to all the individuals I have met and cared for during my years as a physician. Much knowledge and wisdom has been obtained through our daily interactions. You have put your trust in me and I thank you for the opportunity to care for you.

Robert H. Sorensen, M.D.

Acknowledgments

My special thanks to my wife, Annie, for her countless hours of hard work, dedication and love. And thank you for providing the drawings within the text of the book.

Additionally, I would like to thank Sherry LaPorte for the cover design of Why Do I Wheeze? as well as her numerous artistic contributions to the North Shore Asthma Clinic.

To Kellen, Kate and Maddie-Words cannot express the joy you bring to life. I celebrate you and I love you. -Dad

PREFACE

Why Do I Wheeze? is written for individuals with asthma as well as for the parents and family members of asthmatics. The book is intended to be a resource for education about asthma. The text describes what asthma is, how it affects one's life and physical well being, as well as, appropriate interventions and therapies.

Understanding asthma is essential to its control. In today's world of managed care, doctors' spend little time explaining how, when and why. After completing this book, the reader will be a more informed medical consumer. The information provided will allow for better communication between doctor and patient.

Why Do I Wheeze? is not written to promote any one treatment over another. This book is written to provide the medical consumer with a knowledge base that will ultimately lead to improved health care. Consult with a physician for further evaluation and treatment as needed.

Table of Contents

Dedication...iii

Acknowledgements..v

Preface..vii

What is Asthma?...1

What Does Asthma Feel Like?...................................5

What Causes Asthma?...9

Food Allergy and Asthma..16

Occupational Asthma..17

Testing for Asthma..19

The Emergency Department: 21
When To Go, What to Expect

Asthma Medications...26

Metered Dose Inhalers..34

Assessing Asthma Severity: 36
The Peak Flow Meter

Commonly Asked Questions...................................39

Glossary..62

Appendix...65

WHAT IS ASTHMA?

Asthma is a disease that affects the air passageways of the lungs. The air passageways, called bronchioles, become smaller in size when affected by asthma. This results in much less air flowing into and out of the lung with each breath causing the sensation of shortness of breath.

A brief lesson in anatomy of the lungs as well as commonly used terms in asthma is required for a better understanding of how asthma affects the airway.

When you inhale, air passes from the mouth or nose through the vocal cords and into the main 'windpipe' of the lung, called the trachea. (See Figure 1.) The end of the trachea divides into two smaller airways called the left and right bronchi. Subsequently, the air passageways continue to divide at their ends resulting in hundreds of smaller bronchial airways. The bronchial airways are what is affected in asthma. The airways eventually end at the alveoli. The alveoli are the site where oxygen and carbon dioxide are exchanged to and from the blood, respectively.

The bronchial airways are round and covered by muscles that can squeeze the airway and make it smaller or relax completely and make it larger. When the muscles squeeze the airway, it is called bronchospasm. When the muscles relax, it is called bronchodilation. Another term, bronchoconstriction, refers to a smaller airway size that may result from bronchospasm, inflammation or both.

Inflammation is a bodily process that typically occurs as a result of some sort of injury to a part of the body. Inflammation is designed to help heal and protect, however, when it becomes excessive, it can do more harm than good.

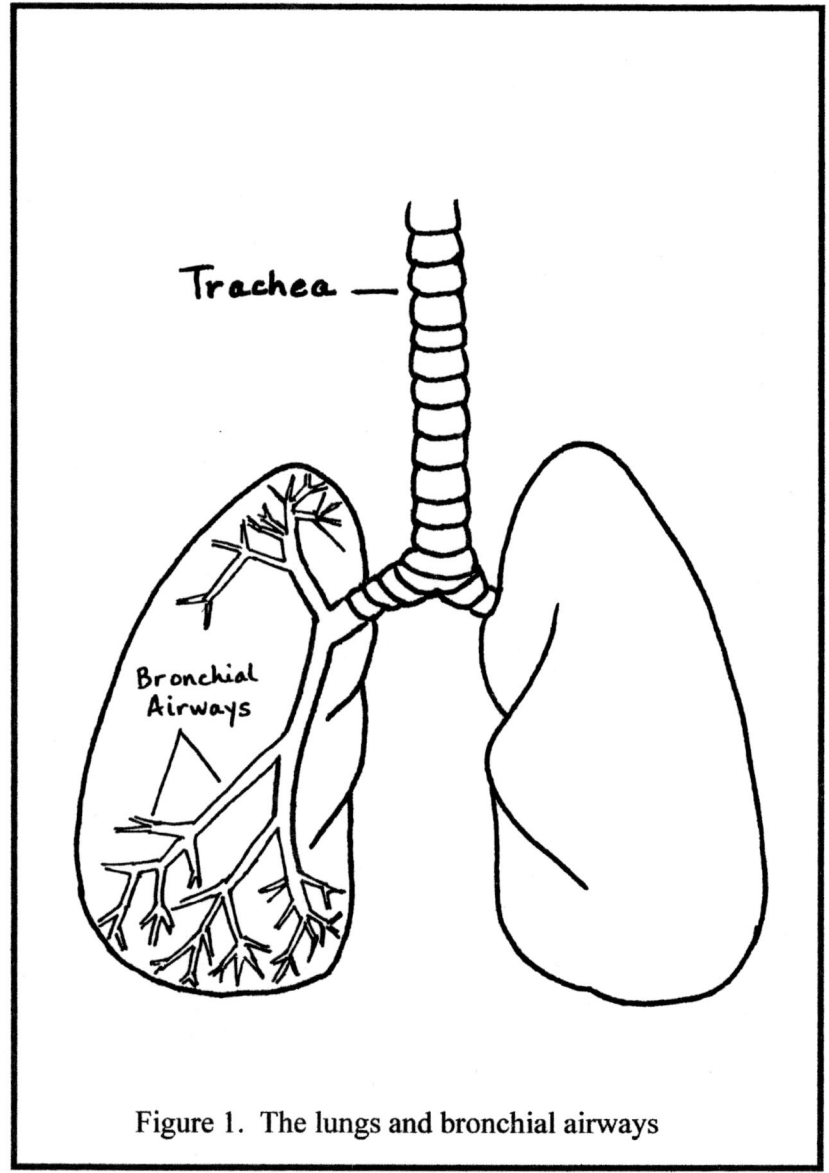

Figure 1. The lungs and bronchial airways

Why Do I Wheeze?

Whenever the body suffers an injury or perceives something is present that doesn't belong, it responds by swelling with fluid. The fluid contains white blood cells that often help to fight infection but also are major contributors to inflammation. The white blood cells secrete fluid containing chemicals that can aid in repair of injury, or, unfortunately, when excessive, may cause scarring or permanent damage to the area instead.

Inflammation of the bronchial airway can be triggered by several mechanisms. This may include direct contact with offending substances or it may occur indirectly from irritation somewhere else in the body. When the airway becomes inflamed, there is increased blood flow, secretion of chemicals into the airway, swelling, and thus, narrowing of the airway. This may also trigger bronchospasm. This illustrates the importance of treating inflammation in asthma, rather than just treating bronchospasm.

Other examples of inflammation that you may be more familiar with include: 1. Swelling and excessive fluid secretion of the nose and eyes when triggered by hayfever allergy or, similarly, the common cold; 2. Facial swelling with a tooth infection; 3. Skin swelling and redness following an insect sting; 4. Swollen joints from arthritis or following an injury, such as, a twisted ankle. Inflammation is a common response to injury or insult throughout the body. It is an important component of asthma that must not be overlooked nor underestimated when treating asthma.

Inflammation does not resolve rapidly. As you may have experienced, a common head cold can leave you coughing for weeks even though your body's immune system has completely removed the virus. Ankle sprains can seem to keep swelling even though the injury occurred three weeks earlier. Inflammation in the bronchial airway, when left untreated, can result in persistent swelling of the airway as well as scarring. If left untreated long enough, the narrowed airway becomes resistant to bronchodilation and air movement in and out of the lung becomes much less than normal. This results in chronic shortness of breath.

The development of inflammation in the airway varies from person to person. Each individual may respond differently to any given factor that causes asthma. It is known that continuous or repeated exposure to factors causing asthma can lead to chronic inflammatory changes in the airway that may not be reversible. To use an analogy, imagine a water pipe that continually has highly mineralized water going through it. Eventually, the minerals begin to adhere to the pipe and the flow of water through the pipe is decreased. The pipe must be cleaned thoroughly or replaced to increase water flow. In the bronchial airway, we can 'clean' it with proper medications early on, but, without treatment, it will have to be replaced.

In summary, asthma is a disease of the bronchial airway. It results from the narrowing of the airway by bronchospasm, inflammation, or both. As the airway becomes smaller in size, it becomes more difficult to pass air in and out of the lungs and the affected individual becomes short of breath. The usual ease of breathing now becomes work and each breath requires extra effort. **Successful treatment of asthma must be directed at prevention, with reduced exposure to those factors that trigger asthma, control of inflammation and relief of bronchospasm.**

WHAT DOES ASTHMA FEEL LIKE?

The individual with asthma will describe many different feelings. Shortness of breath or air hunger is very common. Most often, people state they just can't get a good breath in. This is a constant sensation and often provokes anxiety. Some individuals describe the sensation as a tight hug that limits their ability to breathe in effectively. Others may complain of chronic cough or chest congestion. "If I could just get this phlegm up, I know I would feel better." Still, others describe a fullness to their lower chest or upper abdomen, similar to eating too much. Children may say nothing at all or may complain that their chest hurts. Their limited vocabulary or general knowledge may not allow for an accurate description of what they are feeling. This is where a parent needs to pay close attention to their child's behavior and actions, in order to give an examining physician the best idea of what has been happening.

The shortness of breath of asthma can come on rapidly, in a matter of seconds, or, gradually, over hours or days. When the shortness of breath is not relieved quickly, the 'work' of breathing becomes much harder. The diaphragm muscle located under the lung normally contracts to pull air into the lung. Individuals with asthma symptoms use additional muscles in their chest and neck to help lift the rib cage in order to get more air into the lung. These muscles provide important extra help for the asthmatic, but, they will become tired and sore if used for a prolonged attack of asthma. Individuals recovering from prolonged shortness of breath will often complain of chest heaviness and soreness despite being able to breathe better. This is just like your muscles feel after starting a new exercise program. If they are not trained regularly, there can be a lot of muscle aches the next day or two.

Nocturnal asthma refers to the narrowing of the bronchial

airway that occurs during sleep. This is a common problem in many asthmatics that often goes unrecognized. Nocturnal asthma may not be noticed due to sleep. Individuals may have restless sleep, cough, wheezing or severe shortness of breath that goes unrecognized until waking during the night or early morning. Frequently, spouses often here the signs of nocturnal asthma and will wake their partner to advise them of the need for rescue medication.

The causes of nocturnal asthma are no different than other forms of asthma. Prevention of nocturnal asthma requires all the usual appropriate treatments for asthma care. Additionally, patients may receive a medication specific for nocturnal asthma. Serevent®, is a medication that, when inhaled, acts to open the bronchial airway by relaxing the surrounding muscles. Serevent® does not work immediately, rather, it works slowly, over a prolonged period of time, usually longer than most sleep time duration. It has no value for the treatment of an acute attack of asthma. If an acute attack of asthma occurs during the night, after you have used Serevent®, then you will need to use your regular rescue medication. Serevent® may also be used during the day, helping to prevent or lessen the severity of other episodes of asthma.

Asthma symptoms can be intermittent or constant. The shortness of breath associated with asthma can come on quickly after exposure to substances or activities that provoke it or it can come on gradually and persist for days, weeks or months if left untreated. Asthma can become severe and life threatening at any time, regardless of duration.

When asthma comes on quickly, it is usually due to bronchospasm. There may or may not be inflammation in the airway. This varies for each individual based on the duration and severity of their asthma. The rapid onset of shortness of breath after recent exposure (few seconds to minutes) to a triggering agent is called the "immediate" or "early" asthmatic response.

A delayed response to a triggering agent can occur hours or

days following exposure. This is called the "late phase" asthmatic response. It also involves bronchospasm of the bronchial airway, but, more importantly, it probably signals the development of inflammation in the airway. The shortness of breath associated with this "late phase" response may be less than, equal to or greater than an early response. Often, the shortness of breath is gradual, perhaps not as noticeable, and may not be as easy to treat as the early phase. Both rescue medication and anti-inflammatory medication is required. Additionally, an individual with chronic asthma and inflammation can have an "immediate" response to the appropriate trigger. This can result in a life threatening asthma attack. Thus, the importance of early treatment and prevention of all asthma symptoms cannot be over emphasized.

Additionally, those individuals with persistent shortness of breath despite treatment, may lose the ability to realize how short of breath they are. They gradually change their lifestyle, decrease their activity level and begin to forget how short of breath they are. A similar example would be putting on tight pants. You know they are tight when you put them on, but, after an hour or so, you don't notice the tightness so much. You become used to it.

The chronically ill asthmatic has much less reserve lung space or functioning bronchial airway. The airway is narrowed from bronchospasm and inflammation, or, completely blocked by inflammatory fluid and cells. Often, this blockage will dry out to form a solid plug that prevents further passage of air or medication. When a few airways become blocked, the breathing becomes much more difficult. Any sudden trigger may cause increased bronchospasm with devastating consequences.

This loss of sensation to shortness of breath is not uncommon. Individuals are frequently evaluated in the emergency room for shortness of breath and complain of just being a little worse, when, in fact, they are using only 30-40% of their entire lung to breathe. This makes objective assessment of asthma important. This can be accomplished with the use of a peak flow meter. This is a simple, lightweight, plastic device that measures how fast you can blow air out of your lungs. Just blow into the mouthpiece as hard and fast as you can, then read the meter on the side. The result is compared to a standardized measurement for age and height. This will be covered at length later in the text.

If you have ever suffered from shortness of breath, regardless of the cause, you are probably well aware of these feelings. The shortness of breath from asthma may occur gradually or rapidly. At times you may worry that you will never get another breath in. When this happens, it is important to try and stay calm and avoid any strenuous activity other than breathing. Use your medications as directed and if you do not improve rapidly, or continue to get worse, seek immediate medical attention or call 911 for assistance.

Finally, if you don't have asthma but want to know what it feels like, try this simple test. Do not attempt this if you are not in excellent health. Take a drinking straw and purse your lips around one end. Now set a timer for five minutes, pinch your nose completely shut and start breathing through the straw. Pay close attention to your body over time. Note how you have to breathe more often and how, eventually, your chest is moving to help you get more air in with each breath. Had enough, imagine this sensation lasting for hours or days with the associated anxiety and frustration it causes.

WHAT CAUSES ASTHMA?

The causes of asthma are diverse. While allergy is often thought to be the main cause of asthma, there are many other factors involved in the development and progression of the disease. Furthermore, it is important to realize that we have not yet identified all the causes of asthma. Identifying the exact cause(s) of asthma is not always possible, making daily treatment with preventive medications essential to the control of asthma.

Allergy to pollen, house dust, house-dust mites, animal dander, and mold spores are common causes of asthma. The term allergy refers to an individual developing sensitivity or immunity to a substance through previous contact. This is a reaction of the immune system. After exposure to a particular substance, for example, pollen, the body's immune system may recognize it as a foreign invader that must be removed or isolated to prevent harm. In allergic individuals, this reaction between the immune system and the triggering agent or allergen, results in the release of chemicals that trigger the allergic reaction. For pollen, itchy watery eyes, sneezing and a runny nose may occur. If the reaction is more severe, shortness of breath and wheezing may result. Allergic reactions can occur immediately after exposure to a triggering substance or they may be delayed for several hours after exposure. This delayed response, which may occur hours after leaving the source of the reaction can make its identification as the triggering agent more difficult.

House-dust mites are microscopic insects that eat dead skin as it is shed from the body of people or animals. They will also eat the scales from hair, also known as dander. The digestive waste of the mite contains potential allergens. As the name implies, house-dust mites and house-dust mite allergen are found in house dust. House dust collects everywhere and mites are found in high concentrations in bedding, stuffed toys and furniture as well as carpeting. They prefer to live in a warm, humid environment. The house dust mite is considered to be a significant cause of asthma.

The mite population can be controlled but not completely eliminated. Mattresses and pillows should be encased with mite resistant covers. Bedding materials and sleepwear should be washed in hot water, at least 140°F. Synthetic or cotton blankets are preferable to wool. Bare floors (wood, tile, vinyl) are preferable to carpet. Use throw rugs that are washable. Leather, vinyl or wood furniture is preferred over fabric covered stuffed furniture. Try to limit the number of stuffed toys available for play. Ideally, buy washable stuffed toys. Finally, if you have any pets with hair, keep them out of the bedroom. The shedding of hair or skin acts as a stimulus for a mite population explosion.

Animal allergy is another cause of asthma. Cat allergy is reported to cause more asthma than dog allergy. Other common pet allergies include: gerbils; rabbits; guinea pigs; and pet mice. This list could include almost anything.

Removing a family pet can be devastating. However, at times, it is the only option to regain control of asthma symptoms. If this is not an option, then it is important to isolate the pet from the bedroom and frequent play areas. It is important to stress that this latter procedure may be of no benefit whatsoever! It has been demonstrated that cat allergens remain in the home for up to six months after cat removal, despite what is considered adequate cleaning of floors, walls and linens. Individuals with frequent asthma symptoms from exposure to pets should give every consideration to pet removal from the home. Prolonged contact with these allergens may lead to chronic changes or scarring in the lung that could result in long term disability from asthma.

Recently, substances in cockroach feces have been found to be a trigger for asthma in some individuals. One need not play with cockroaches to develop this allergy. The presence of roaches in a house may go undetected as they are typically out and about only at night. Placing roach traps in a bedroom or kitchen may help to identify infestation. The most appropriate course of action is a thorough cleaning of the area and utilization of proper insecticide. This should not be sprayed with the asthmatic individual in the house. Spray a bedroom early in the morning and air the room out so the insecticide does not trigger any symptoms. Make sure food is cleaned up and stored properly in sealed containers. Do not allow any food of any kind in the bedroom.

Another substance known to trigger asthma symptoms is mold. Mold is a term used to describe the growth of fungus on decaying material or areas that are rich in moisture. Many individuals are sensitive to mold spores that are released as the fungus grows. Mold is found both inside and outside the house. Routine weather reports on television will often give a pollen and mold spore count. These are usually elevated in spring and autumn. Sensitive individuals may suffer from sneezing, itch, watery eyes, and asthma. Mold grows in your house as well. It can be found in dark, moist places like the basement, or wherever water accumulates. The humidifier on a forced air furnace may have standing water over the summer months which can promote the growth of mold. The filter on the humidifier should be changed prior to winter use of the furnace. Potted plants and soil within the house is another potential source of mold.

Smoke in any form can be hazardous to people with asthma. Cigar and cigarette smoke contains many chemicals that may trigger bronchospasm or bronchial inflammation. Smoke from the fireplace or wood burning stove may also worsen symptoms. Obviously, smoke is to be avoided. No smoking should be allowed in the home of an asthmatic. The idea of smoking in one room that is not visited by the asthmatic is not enough to prevent exposure and subsequent symptoms.

Upper respiratory infection is a common trigger for asthma. It may be the initial cause of asthma is some cases. Additionally, many asthmatics will routinely have more asthma symptoms when the have a cold or bronchitis.

The common cold is caused by a variety of viruses. These

viruses infect the tissues of the nose, sinuses and back of the throat. Inflammation of the nose and sinuses is a well known trigger for asthma. It is not known why inflammation in this area causes asthma, but, many theories abound. Typically, the asthma resulting from a cold develops over days, shortness of breath becomes progressively worse and does not respond completely to the use of rescue medication. Antibiotics are of no value during this kind of viral infection. If fluid accumulates in the sinuses, a bacterial infection could occur, and antibiotics may be necessary for improvement. Additionally, sinusitis, or inflammation of the sinuses, can be caused by allergy alone. This can resemble infection with thick creamy secretions, but, will not respond well to antibiotics.

The sinuses are open spaces within the skull. They have holes that allow them to drain fluid into the nasal cavity. When inflammation and swelling occur, the sinuses do not drain well. The holes may become plugged, fluid accumulates and provides a rich broth for bacteria to grow in. Bacterial sinusitis is often associated with headache, facial pain, tooth pain and fever. When this occurs, it is important to get the sinuses to drain. If the fluid is gone, the number of bacteria in the sinus is greatly decreased and the infection may resolve spontaneously. Topical decongestant nasal sprays may be used for up to 3 days to promote drainage. An ice pack to the face for twenty minutes several times a day may be helpful, if not soothing. Over-the-counter decongestant remedies may be helpful, but, send medication throughout your body for a localized problem.

Sinusitis is often a chronic problem. Inflammation of the sinuses is a similar process to inflammation of the bronchial airway. When the nasal airway is also affected, and it usually is, it is called rhinosinusitis. This can be caused by infection or allergy. Again, for reasons unknown, sinus inflammation causes worsening of asthma in some individuals. The important point to remember is that this inflammation, like the inflammation of asthma must be treated effectively. This is a common omission by physicians managing asthma patients. The patient may receive the appropriate anti-inflammatory medicine for their asthma without treating the primary cause in the nose and sinuses.

The bronchial airways of the lung can also become infected with viruses and bacteria. This can result in bronchospasm and inflammation. In young children, an infection with Respiratory Syncytial Virus (RSV) can often be the cause of the first episode of wheezing. Some medical professionals believe this virus promotes inflammation of the bronchial airway leading to chronic asthma. Each individual responds differently to infection with this virus and not everyone wheezes from it. Children born prematurely or with chronic lung problems tend to suffer more severe symptoms with this infection. Medication is available to fight this virus, but, is utilized in only the most severe cases. A simple test can be performed at most hospital labs for RSV. A small sample of nasal secretions is all that is required. Work continues on a vaccine against RSV.

Influenza virus can also worsen asthma. Individuals, including children, with asthma, are strongly urged to receive an annual vaccination against influenza in the mid to late fall. Influenza, or flu, typically involves a sore throat, runny nose, high fever, body aches and a non-productive cough. Symptoms may last 7-10 days. Newer medications are available to fight the flu. They must be taken in the first 48 hours of symptoms. Typically, they may shorten the course of the disease by 1-2 days or so. Individuals with asthma that become infected with influenza may note increasing shortness of breath, frequent wheezing or chest tightness. As always, utilize rescue medication and have a complete evaluation by a qualified physician.

Mycoplasma is the name of a bacteria that has been found in the bronchial airway of individuals with asthma. This bacteria is a well known cause of pneumonia and is believed to be a cause of chronic inflammation of the bronchial airway when left untreated. This infection can be adequately treated with antibiotics such as erythromycin or tetracycline. The inflammation may take weeks or months to resolve. At this time there are no rapid or easy tests that confirm this type of infection. Frequently, physicians may initiate treatment based on history and physical exam for a presumed mycoplasma infection.

The previously described infections frequently worsen asthma symptoms. The shortness of breath becomes gradually worse and often results in a visit to a physician for evaluation and breathing treatments. Many physicians are aware of this phenomenon in their asthmatic patients and will often prescribe a steroid medication, such as prednisone, at the first sign of infection. Steroid medications slow down the development of inflammation. This results in less inflammation in the bronchial airway than might otherwise occur with infection. Overall, shortness of breath will not be as bad or will improve more rapidly than without treatment. If your asthma worsens with infection, talk to your doctor about getting medication to use at the first sign of an upper respiratory infection. This preventive technique works well in both children and adults.

Another cause of asthma symptoms that is often overlooked is gastroesophageal reflux disease, also referred to as GERD. This refers to stomach acid and/or food being flushed from the stomach up into the esophagus where it causes irritation and eventually, inflammation and scarring of the esophagus. It is believed that the irritation of the esophagus by stomach acid can lead to asthma symptoms. It may be related to acid stimulating nerves in the esophagus which send a signal to the brain. In turn, the brain sends a signal to the bronchial airway to constrict or close down because some acid might leak in if it gets up by the opening of the trachea. Additionally, it may be that the airway is responding directly to acid fumes that reach the back of the throat and are subsequently inhaled. Other mechanisms may exist that result in asthma from GERD that are not yet identified.

Reflux of acid occurs for a variety of reasons. It can occur in infants, especially those that are born prematurely. This may be related to a lack of strength in the muscles that usually _ _ the esophagus closed from the stomach. Adults are also affected. The symptoms of reflux are variable. Some individuals may have no symptoms whatsoever while others will complain of indigestion or a brackish taste in the back of the mouth.

Reflux can be treated effectively with medications and alteration in diet. Weight loss may be necessary for the obese. Occasionally, in severe cases, surgery is required for improvement. Despite adequate treatment of reflux, asthma symptoms may persist for months and must continue to be treated with appropriate medications.

Have you ever seen a child stop running at a soccer game after five minutes and they're gasping for air? They stop running and walk up and down the field. This may represent exercise induced asthma or EIA. It may occur without a previous history of asthma or it may occur in anyone with a history of asthma. EIA generally begins within a few minutes after the increased activity begins. EIA may get better with rest, may resolve despite continued activity or may need to be treated with rescue medication. There are several medications available for EIA. In general, the inhaled medications must be used between ten and thirty minutes prior to the onset of increased activity.

EIA is just one reason for being short of breath with exercise. Lack of physical conditioning will also result in shortness of breath but should not result in wheezing unless the individual also has EIA. Heart disease may also cause shortness of breath with increased activity and may be associated with wheezing. Consult your physician to determine why you're short of breath with exercise.

Exposure to cold air can trigger bronchospasm in sensitive individuals. This is not an allergic reaction. The mechanism by which cold air causes this problem is unknown. Typically, temperatures near or below freezing will trigger bronchospasm. Like exercise induced asthma, cold air induced asthma can be prevented by medication used shortly before exposure. Prompt relief can also be obtained with rescue medication. Make sure the canister of the inhaler is warmed to room temperature prior to use. Do not use a cold inhaler.

FOOD ALLERGY AND ASTHMA

Food allergy refers to symptoms resulting from a specific reaction of the immune system to a specific food protein. The body organs that are most often affected by food allergy include the skin, gastrointestinal tract and the respiratory system. The foods that affect children most frequently include eggs, milk, peanuts, soy, wheat, tree nuts, fish and shellfish. Adults are most sensitive to peanuts, tree nuts, shellfish and fish. Food related asthma is much more common in children than adults. A history of recurrent wheezing is a sensitive indicator for allergy when it occurs with repeated exposure to the same food allergens. Skin and blood testing for allergy may be helpful, although, some individuals may test positive for allergy yet tolerate eating that same substance regularly. Others may test negative, yet, react to the same food every time. Often, a food challenge, eating the suspected substance, in a controlled setting such as the doctor's office, is necessary to prove an association between food and asthma, safely. Additionally, it should be noted that the aroma of some foods or vapors from cooking, may trigger asthma symptoms in sensitive individuals.

Anaphylaxis, a severe allergic reaction manifested by very low blood pressure, hives, lightheadedness and shortness of breath may occur immediately following ingestion of a triggering agent or may occur after a brief delay in time. This is often a life threatening event that requires immediate medical attention. Individuals with a history of similar reactions should carry medication to treat this. Adrenaline, also called epinephrine, is essential to treat anaphylaxis. It is available in a special syringe that will automatically inject the correct dose when applied firmly to the arm or thigh. Medical attention must be sought after injection as the reaction may recur within minutes. Nuts and shellfish are the most common cause of anaphylaxis from food allergy.

OCCUPATIONAL ASTHMA

Asthma symptoms brought on by exposure to a substance(s) at work that is not typically found outside of work defines occupational asthma. The diagnosis of occupational asthma requires that shortness of breath be directly related to being at work. This association can be difficult to prove. For example, someone may be sensitive to something at work, but, may not develop shortness of breath until hours after leaving work. As sensitivity or hyperreactivity of the bronchial airway increases, symptoms may come on more rapidly after exposure to the triggering agent. Others will develop shortness of breath within minutes of exposure. Additionally, individuals with a previous history of asthma may develop worsening symptoms at work from a substance unique to the workplace. This too, is occupational asthma.

The diagnosis of occupational asthma should only be made when exposure to the workplace brings on symptoms of asthma associated with an objective measurement of decreased airflow. This is accomplished by measuring peak flow rates or other spirometric tests of lung function, before, during and after work. If there is a significant decrease in airflow measured, then a rescue medication should be administered and any measurable improvement documented.

Occupational asthma frequently improves while on vacation or over a weekend off. Improvement may be slow, but, some people note that they feel great on Monday morning and are out of breath by the end of the day. This chronology is often the first clue to the diagnosis of occupational asthma.

It is important to remember that repeated exposure to a triggering agent or allergen can lead to chronic shortness of breath that worsens over time. Eventually, the ability to reverse the inflammation and bronchospasm may decrease. Thus, emphasis on avoidance and prevention cannot be over stressed.

Additionally, specialized testing for some workplace substances may be available by an allergist, pulmonary specialist or occupational health physician. This can help to identify triggering agents and thus allow for specific alterations in workplace exposure.

The diagnosis of occupational asthma carries significant implications for both employee and employer. Obviously, serious complications of asthma in the workplace can lead to long term disability and in the most serious instance, death. The affected employee should first seek medical care for acute symptoms of asthma. This should be followed by reporting of symptoms and required treatment to the employer. Every effort must be made to avoid potential exposure. This may require doing a different activity at work, or, in some cases, changing jobs. Just moving from one department to the next may not be enough. Exposures may be less, but symptoms may still occur. Common occupations associated with asthma are listed on the next page.

Grain dust, grain dust mites	Farmers, grain storage worker
Fowl mites	Poultry workers
Urine, danders	Animal handlers
Henna (dye)	Hair dresser
Drugs, enzymes	Pharmaceutical workers
Latex	Health care workers, glove makers
Dyes, wool	Textile workers
Western red cedar, oak, African maple	Woodworkers, carpenters, sawmill workers
Diisocyanates	Plastics, polyurethane producers, spray painters, roofers
Beans	Food processors, farmers, longshoremen, fertilizer workers
Flour	Bakers, flour mill workers
Shellfish	Food processors
Glutaraldehyde, Formaldehyde	Healthcare workers
Vegetable gums	Printer, hairdresser, carpet makers

REACTIVE AIRWAY DYSFUNCTION SYNDROME – RADS

Don't be intimidated by the big words, this is asthma by a different name and a different cause. According to the definition of RADS, the affected individual must have had a high level irritant exposure, usually resulting from a single major industrial accident. Symptoms typically develop within hours of exposure and do not resolve with rescue medication as well as asthma symptoms from other causes. Some individuals may not develop symptoms immediately, but, will with repeated exposures. RADS resulting from workplace exposure is considered a form of occupational asthma. Common causes include chlorine gas, sulfuric acid, ammonia and acute smoke inhalation.

Inflammation is found in the airway early in the course of the disease. Treatment includes use of anti-inflammatory medications and bronchodilators. With appropriate treatment, symptoms will often resolve over a four to six month period without any residual problems. If left untreated, bronchial airway scarring could occur, leading to chronic shortness of breath.

TESTING FOR ASTHMA

Is there a good test for asthma? This is not an easy question to answer. There is a test that is used occasionally, called a methacholine challenge test. The patient inhales a drug, methacholine, and the test is considered positive for asthma if the patient's ability to rapidly exhale is diminished by 20%, when compared to the same ability prior to inhaling the drug. Like all testing in medicine and science, the test is not perfect. The test will accurately identify some people with asthma. However, sometimes the test may be falsely positive (someone without asthma is diagnosed with asthma) or falsely negative (someone with asthma is told they don't have asthma). Similarly, testing for exercise induced asthma before and after increased activity may not adequately reflect the actual shortness of breath associated with exercise.

The same problems can be encountered with allergy testing. Scratch testing, intradermal injection (into the skin) of allergens and specialized blood testing for specific allergies can indicate sensitivity in some individuals. Yet, when exposed, they may have no reaction. Similarly, others may test negative for allergy,

yet, react immediately when exposed to the allergen in question.
Should you be tested for asthma and allergy? If you feel short of breath, wheeze or cough a lot, and get better with rescue medication, then you don't need asthma testing. If a doctor examined and treated you for asthma, and your symptoms have occurred on a few or more occasions, then you probably have asthma. Testing for asthma will not offer any more to your diagnosis.

Allergy testing may be helpful in identifying triggering agents, when the test is accurate. Identification allows for removal of causative agents which may result in improvement in symptoms. However, other agents may go unidentified, and thus, symptoms may persist.

Do allergy shots help asthma get better? There is a great deal of controversy about the value of allergy shots. Allergy shots involve giving small doses of known allergens into the skin. This helps to regulate the immune system and tries to make it less sensitive to allergens. This has never been convincingly demonstrated to improve asthma symptoms with the possible exception of treatment for dust mite allergen. Additionally, it is important to note that individuals with moderate to severe chronic asthma should not receive allergy injections because of the risk of a severe, life threatening asthma attack.

THE EMERGENCY DEPARTMENT: WHEN TO GO, WHAT TO EXPECT

The hospital emergency room and outpatient acute care centers provide emergency treatment for shortness of breath. The decision to seek medical care may be difficult for various reasons: transportation problems; prior obligations; feeling that you might get better in a short while; or fear of doctors and hospitals. The best reason to go is to breathe better and easier and to avoid the serious complications of asthma. Remember, the sooner you go, the sooner you'll be better. When should you seek medical evaluation? Some guidelines are listed below.

1. If you think for one second you should see a physician, then go.
2. If you use your rescue medication (bronchodilator) and do not improve rapidly, then go.
3. If you can't say more than two or three words at a time without stopping to breathe, then go.
4. If your peak flow rate is less than 60% of your personal best, then go.
5. If you feel anxious while short of breath, then go.
6. If your child is wheezing, can't stop coughing, can't talk, or the skin between their ribs gets "pulled in" while breathing, then go.
7. If you feel tired because you are "working hard" and using your chest and neck muscles to help you breathe, then go.
8. If you have chronic asthma with daily symptoms that are getting worse, then go.
9. If you are short of breath and have ever been admitted as an inpatient to a hospital for asthma and your symptoms are worse, you should go.
10. If you have asthma symptoms that are getting progressively worse over several days, then you should go.

How should you travel to the doctor? The quickest way is to call for an ambulance. The advantage of the ambulance is, that most often, the personnel are skilled in the assessment of asthma and can start treatment immediately. Otherwise, have someone drive you. If you can't talk for very long or are struggling to breathe, call the ambulance, not a friend. Remember, your symptoms may be distracting to you or someone driving you and this could cause an accident with associated injuries.

What can you expect after you arrive at the emergency

department? First, if you arrive without the assistance of an ambulance, you'll need to let someone know that you are short of breath from asthma. Go directly to the receptionist or triage nurse when you arrive and tell them you are very short of breath. The staff is trained to respond to these words and should take you back for immediate evaluation and treatment. They should not ask you to sit down and fill out paper work. If they do, then tell them you are too ill to do it immediately and would prefer to be immediately evaluated. They need to know that you are in distress.

Your initial evaluation should include measurement of your pulse rate, breathing rate, blood pressure, temperature and oxygen saturation. Your oxygen saturation is measured by a device called a pulse oximeter. It painlessly fits on fingers, toes or ear lobes. It gives a measurement of how much oxygen is bound to your red blood cells. This can be helpful in monitoring your condition as it gets better or worse. Ideally, a peak flow measurement should be obtained prior to therapy. However, this may not be possible for those individuals that are severely short of breath. Peak flow rate is useful to objectively measure the response to treatment. Several peak flow rates may be obtained during a prolonged stay in the emergency department. Some physicians may choose to use physical examination and the patient's subjective feelings of improvement or worsening to determine the response to therapy instead of repeat peak flow measurements. Evaluation and treatment may be initiated by the nursing staff prior to a physician's exam.

Next, you should meet the attending physician. The physician should ask detailed questions concerning your current problems, daily medications, as well as past medical problems. If you can remember, it is always helpful to bring all your medications with you, including any over-the-counter medications or herbal drugs. If you are severely short of breath and unable to talk, the interview will obviously be curtailed to yes and no questions to which you may nod the answer.

Parents should always accompany children, including older teenagers. Many children are poor historians or unwilling to answer questions that may be crucial to proper treatment.

The interview and physical exam may occur at the same time when the patient is in obvious distress. A thorough exam includes examination of the nose, mouth and neck, as well as, listening to the lungs and heart. Examination of the lungs should be repeated during the course of treatment. Every physician will have his favorite way to treat asthma, but, there should be some similarities between all doctors.

Physicians evaluate the severity of asthma through history taking and physical examination. Visual inspection of the asthmatic patient often reveals someone sitting still and obviously "working" to breathe. The stethoscope allows us to hear air flow through the lung. Wheezing, a high pitched whistling noise is often heard with asthma, but, is not always present. Severe, life threatening asthma, may present with a lack of any breath sounds at all. The patient may have a bluish discoloration to the lips or fingernails, cold clammy skin and inability to speak more than one or two words at a time. Additionally, knowing if this attack was sudden or going on for days may make a difference in treatment with certain steroid medication. Remember, you can always give additional information as you remember it or when you can finally talk. Your history often holds the key to proper treatment and may be beneficial in prevention of further episodes or in preventing a relapse of this particular episode. Finally, the physician should explain how he/she plans to treat you. Ask questions if you are unsure of anything.

The main treatment throughout the United States for more than ten years has been the administration of "beta" medicines by inhalation. "Beta" refers to a type of receptor in the bronchial airway that the medicine binds to. This results in a chemical reaction that causes the muscle around the airway to relax followed by increased airflow in and out of the lung. Think of the medicine as a key that opens a lock (the receptor).

Beta medicines are most often administered by nebulizer. This is a device that circulates air or oxygen through a solution of medicine. The solution becomes aerosolized and the patient breathes in the mist, delivering medication directly to the bronchial airways. The beta medicine can also be administered by a metered dose inhaler. It takes 10-20 puffs from an inhaler to approximate the dose in one nebulizer treatment. Additionally, beta medicines are available for injection. Repeated nebulizations are often necessary for significant improvement.

Inhaled medication will be much less effective in those individuals that are not moving much air in and out of the lung. These are the sickest patients and require careful observation and repeated examinations. These patients are best treated with injected medications such as adrenaline (also called epinephrine) or terbutaline. These medications may also be administered multiple times until the patient improves significantly. Oxygen therapy is often required as well.

Many asthmatics will respond quickly to treatment and be discharged home without further difficulties. Others will require multiple treatments and be in the emergency room for hours before a decision is made to send them home or admit them to the hospital.

Anyone requiring multiple treatments or for those with increasing symptoms over several days should receive anti-inflammatory steroid medication during their emergency room visit. Additionally, at discharge to home, either from the emergency room or inpatient hospital bed, each patient treated with steroids should receive a prescription for at least an additional five days of steroid therapy.

This steroid therapy is important for both child and adult asthma patients. The usual medications are prednisone or prednisolone. This can be administered by tablet or syrup. Steroids are given by injection when patients are vomiting or so short of breath that breathing cannot be interrupted to swallow a pill. Overall, there is no difference in effectiveness between injected and swallowed medication.

Finally, when you are told you will be discharged from the emergency room to home, you should feel much better, be breathing easier, have much less anxiety, and be able to talk in full sentences without stopping to breathe. Additionally, you should be able to demonstrate a significant improvement in peak flow measurements compared to flow at the time of your initial assessment. Your chest may hurt or feel heavy if you have been straining to breathe for several hours. This is normal and will improve in a couple of days. You should have access to rescue medication (beta medicine) at the time of discharge. This could be an inhaler, syrup or tablets. As mentioned above, oral steroids are also an integral part of the continued treatment of asthma symptoms after the initial therapy. If the visit and instructions are intimidating, stop and ask questions. Be sure you are fully instructed on the use of inhalers and peak flow meters. Schedule a follow up appointment with your doctor as soon as possible. If you do not have a doctor, ask the emergency staff to recommend a physician for follow up and be sure to get the phone number. Additionally, your insurance company may have a preferred provider they want you to see. Make these calls as soon as possible to avoid delay in follow up and avoid a possible relapse of your condition.

ASTHMA MEDICATIONS

There are multiple medications available to treat asthma. The medications are divided into two groups: anti-inflammatory and rescue medications (bronchodilators). Anti-inflammatory medication is used to actively treat swelling in the bronchial airway as well as to limit and/or prevent inflammation. Bronchodilating medication or rescue medication, treats bronchospasm. These medications are available in multiple forms including: inhaled sprays, mists, powders; tablets and syrups to be taken by mouth; and injections.

ANTI-INFLAMMATORY MEDICATION

The most important point to asthma care will always be prevention. When asthma cannot be prevented, it must be controlled. This control requires anti-inflammatory medication. Currently, there are three classes of medication that prevent or treat the inflammatory process. Consult with your physician to determine which medication is indicated for your condition.

Cromolyn and nedocromil are members of a class of drugs that prevent inflammation by blocking the release of histamine when a triggering agent is encountered. Histamine release is one of the first reactions to occur in the inflammatory process as well as sometimes being associated with sudden onset of bronchospasm. These medications are available for inhalation into the bronchial airway. They must be used daily, regardless of symptom presence or absence, to have any effect. Cromolyn is also available for nasal administration for the symptoms of allergic rhinitis. These medications are for prevention only and do not treat inflammation. They are effective for prevention of exercise induced asthma when taken one half hour prior to onset of increased activity. Side effects are minimal, but, can include bronchospasm in some individuals.

Leukotriene (luke-o-tri-een) inhibitors or blockers are the newest class of anti-inflammatory drugs. These medications are currently available in tablet or chewable tablet form. Children as young as six may use one (Singulair®) of the three currently available medications. Leukotrienes are chemicals secreted by inflammatory cells in the bronchial airway that can cause bronchospasm directly as well as stimulate more swelling and secretions in the airway tissues. This new class of drugs is the first to take specific aim at chemicals known to cause asthma. These medications work by preventing the body from making leukotrienes or by blocking the receptor in the airway where the chemical would bind and stimulate inflammation and bronchospasm. One of the three drugs currently available requires frequent blood tests as it can harm the liver. This is not the same drug that is available for children.

Inhaled steroid medication is considered the drug of choice to prevent and control the symptoms of asthma. However, they are of no immediate value during an acute attack of asthma. Unfortunately, the word steroid is often met with fear or misunderstanding and some individuals will refuse this treatment despite its ability to help control asthma symptoms. Inhaled steroid is available in metered dose inhalers that spray a fine mist as well as in powder form which is inhaled through a special device that accelerates a set amount of powder into the airway when properly utilized. Steroids can also be administered through a small volume nebulizer, but, this is not commonly used at this time.

When using a steroid metered dose inhaler, a spacer device should be used to administer the medication. The spacer is a hollow chamber with a mouthpiece at one end and a slot for the inhaler at the other end. The inhaler mechanism is activated, the mist goes into the chamber and the patient takes several, slow, deep breaths to get the medication into the lung. These spacers have been found to improve drug delivery and to reduce side effects. These potential side effects include a rash around or including the lips, yeast infection of mouth and throat and hoarseness from vocal cord irritation. You should always rinse your mouth with water after using any inhaled steroid medication in order to reduce the risk of yeast infection. It should be emphasized that these side effects are not common and do not outweigh the benefits of inhaled steroid therapy.

Steroids, whether ingested, injected or inhaled, inhibit some of the normal activities of white blood cells that are responsible for the inflammation of asthma. When stimulated by steroids, these white blood cells do not respond to triggering agents as they usually might. Typically, after stimulation by a triggering agent, the white blood cells may secrete multiple chemicals that increase the inflammatory process. Some chemicals will be destructive to normal airway tissues, others will result in bronchospasm (the leukotrienes) while other chemical secretions will act to recruit other inflammatory white blood cells into the bronchial airway. This process becomes repetitive and ultimately destructive to normal lung tissues.

The inflammatory process can occur despite adequate therapy, but, may tend to be less severe and may respond more quickly to large doses of oral steroids if the patient is currently using inhaled steroids. This should result in better breathing and decreased use of rescue medication. Inhaled steroid medication does not work immediately. To control asthma, it must be taken every day, regardless of symptom severity.

There is no discounting the fact that steroids are strong medicines. They can affect the body in many ways. For example, it has been suggested that inhaled steroids are associated with slower growth rates in children. It does not affect final stature. Some studies have failed to show this effect when specifically studied for. Therefore, it may vary between individuals. Additionally, large doses of oral steroids are known to cause a loss of muscle and a gain of fat and sometimes excess water known as edema. This typically occurs after prolonged use. Steroids can also affect the body's ability to make its own steroid, cortisol. This can lead to problems when the body undergoes physical stress, like major surgery. This may actually require additional steroids to make up for the body's deficit. Prolonged use of steroids can lead to diabetes in some individuals and is well known to make blood sugar rise above normal in people already known to be diabetic. Always report current or recent steroid use to any physician you are seeing for any illness, physical or mental.

The oral dosing of steroids is much stronger than the inhaled form and works quickly (within 18-24 hours) to calm inflammation that is progressing rapidly. One should continue to use inhaled steroids while on the oral dose unless otherwise directed by a physician.

Inhaled steroids are beneficial to asthma care. The majority of inhaled medicine goes into the lung where it is metabolized to relatively inactive medication. This is considered beneficial as the remainder of the body receives only negligible amounts of the drug. If you use rescue medication three or more times per week, then you should take anti-inflammatory medication. Consult with your physician.

RESCUE MEDICATIONS
BRONCHODILATORS

The term rescue medication refers to those medications that are used to relieve bronchospasm. The goal of rescue medication is relief from the shortness of breath of asthma. These medications work by causing the muscles around the bronchial airway to relax resulting in a larger diameter of the airway and thus increased airflow. The process of opening up the airway is called bronchodilation and the medicines are called bronchodilators. These are also called "beta" medicines because they bind to the beta receptors in the bronchial airway. Bronchodilators also stimulate "hairs" on some of the cells in the airway. These hairs then brush up secretions and the debris of inflammation out of the airway. Many individuals report increased production of sputum or phlegm with the use of these medications. There are many bronchodilators available. A list is included in the appendix. The most common bronchodilator is albuterol. It is also known as Ventolin® and Proventil®.

Bronchodilators are administered through metered dose inhalers, small volume nebulizers, tablets and syrups as well as by injection. Generally, injection of a bronchodilator is reserved for those individuals with severe asthma. These patients are moving so little air in and out of the lungs that inhaled medicine will not reach the site where it needs to work. Injected medicine can reach the site via the blood stream and act more effectively. As breathing improves, treatment with a nebulizer can be given in addition to the injected medicine. The most commonly injected medications are terbutaline and adrenaline (epinephrine). Because these medications are injected, they travel throughout the body in the blood stream. Side effects become more common when the drugs are administered by injection. These can include heart pounding and racing, tremors or shakes in the hands, and a sensation of being cold.

Metered dose inhalers and small volume nebulizers deliver medication directly to the bronchial airway with less side effects than a drug going throughout the entire body. Small volume nebulizers deliver a large dose of medicine in an aerosolized salt water solution. The salt concentration is the same as the salt concentration of our bodily fluids. This solution is helpful in loosening thickened secretions that may be blocking the airway. This is how most emergency departments deliver asthma medication to their patients. Multiple doses of a metered dose inhaler (20-30 actuations) has the same ability to relieve bronchospasm, but, may not be as effective in loosening thickened secretions. Albuterol is the most commonly used drug for the relief of asthma. It is available in a metered dose inhaler, in solution for nebulization, syrup and tablet form. There are other equally effective rescue medications available.

IPRATROPIUM

Ipratropium (Atrovent®) is another drug that acts as a bronchodilator. It is not a beta medicine. Ipratropium works through a different mechanism. This chemical blocks the effects of acetylcholine, a chemical secreted by nerves in the lung. Acetylcholine tends to cause bronchoconstriction and ipratropium prevents or reverses its effect. It is more commonly used in patients who suffer from emphysema or chronic bronchitis. It works well in asthma but appears to be of no added benefit to beta medicine. There is controversy about its use in the most severe cases of asthma where some physicians believe it may be beneficial when used with beta medicine. This seems unusual given that the patients suffering the most severe of asthma attacks will not benefit from most inhaled medicines due to limited air movement. Ipratropium comes in solution for nebulization as well as a metered dose inhaler. It also comes combined with albuterol in a metered dose inhaler, called Combivent®. Overall, most asthmatic patients do well enough without this medicine. It is mentioned here because you may encounter its use during a visit to the emergency room or it may be recommended by your personal physician.

SALMETEROL

Salmeterol (Serevent®) is a type of bronchodilator that has a slower onset of action than other bronchodilators, but, its activity persists for up to twelve hours. It is a beta medicine, but, should never be used to treat acute asthma symptoms because it does not act quickly enough. This drug is normally taken twice daily, by inhalation, via a metered dose inhaler. It is especially helpful in preventing nocturnal asthma. Daily use often results in decreased use of rescue medication.

Studies suggest that in addition to bronchodilation, this medication may prevent the release of histamine and leukotrienes from inflammatory cells when they come into contact with a triggering agent or allergen. It helps to prevent or diminish both the early and late phase asthmatic response to allergens. It is not a substitute for inhaled steroid medication. Despite its many positive actions, asthma can still worsen during its use. Salmeterol is recommended for ages 12 and over. It can be effective for exercise induced asthma. Patients should not take extra inhalations prior to exercise if they are using the medication on the twice daily basis. If EIA is not prevented, use your regular rescue medication prior to or during exercise as needed.

ANTIHISTAMINES

Antihistamines are often thought of as anti-allergy medication. The antihistamine that most people are familiar with is diphenhydramine, also known as Benadryl®. Antihistamines block the effects of histamine. Hay fever is an example of an allergy that results in the release of histamine from contact with pollens. Histamine causes itchy, watery eyes and nose and sneezing. In severe allergic reactions, histamine can cause hives, low blood pressure and wheezing with severe shortness of breath. This is called an anaphylactic reaction. The release of histamine also leads to the secretion of other chemicals that ultimately may result in inflammation to affected areas.

Using antihistamines to prevent or control asthma is controversial. Some scientific studies have shown improvement in asthma symptoms with antihistamines in addition to other therapies. Diphenhydramine and older antihistamines may not be appropriate because of side effects, especially drowsiness.

Newer antihistamines are less likely to cause drowsiness, last longer, and may be beneficial for some individuals, perhaps, depending on the cause and severity of their asthma. Loratadine (Claritin®) is one such antihistamine. It can be taken by children age 6 and above. Azelastine (Astelin®) is another antihistamine that is available as a nasal spray for allergic symptoms of the nose like hay fever. Its chemical structure is such that it also has anti-inflammatory properties. It may be used in children ages 12 and over. It is not yet available in the United States as a tablet.

Talk to your physician about antihistamine use. This must be individualized for each patient. While these medicines are definitely active as antihistamines, their benefit in helping asthma symptoms remains largely unknown.

THEOPHYLLINE

Theophylline is a drug that has been used for years in the treatment of asthma. It works as a bronchodilator. It is administered orally as a tablet, capsule, pellets called sprinkles and as a liquid. It can also be administered intravenously. The intravenous drug is called aminophylline. Theophylline is mentioned here for historical reasons only. While theophylline does have positive effects in asthma, it offers no advantage over the rescue medications available today. It does offer significant disadvantages from a high rate of side effects. These include nausea, restlessness, headaches, irritability, rapid heartbeat and seizures. The amount of theophylline in the blood must be monitored regularly with specialized testing. The dosage must be changed if the levels are too low or too high. Additionally, the level of this medicine in the blood can be elevated to toxic levels after the ingestion of certain other medications.

If this drug is prescribed for you as part of your asthma therapy, ask your doctor why, and, if there is an alternative medication that might work better.

METERED DOSE INHALERS:
GETTING THE MOST FROM EACH PUFF

The metered dose inhaler is the most common way to deliver medication to the bronchial airway. The inhaler consists of a canister filled with medication and a plastic apparatus with a mouthpiece. The canister is depressed into the apparatus resulting in a discharge of medicine through the mouthpiece.

Both anti-inflammatory medication and rescue medication can be delivered through this device. Metered dose means that each time the inhaler is properly depressed, it releases the same dosage of medication. The medication is released into the air as a fine mist. The mist is then inhaled into the lung. Some of the spray will land on the lips, tongue and back of the mouth, but, when properly done, a good portion of the dose will go into the bronchial airways. The technique for inhalation is extremely important. We will describe two different ways to optimize drug delivery to the bronchial airway.

First, shake the canister to assure contents are well mixed. Next, hold the opening of the mouthpiece one to two inches away from your lips. (Do not put the mouthpiece in your mouth as this results in more medication on the tongue and back of throat due to the speed at which it leaves the canister.) Now, take as deep a breath as possible and then blow as much air as you can out of your lungs. Prior to taking in your next breath, depress the canister. The majority of the mist will go into your mouth at which point you should take a deep breath and hold it for five seconds, then breath normally. Practice this in front of a mirror. You will see the mist suspended in your mouth and can watch it disappear as you breathe in. Wait one minute before taking another dose.

The second method of inhalation involves the use of a spacer device. (See Figure 2.) This is a hollow chamber with a mouthpiece on one end and a hole in the other end for the inhaler. In this technique, you are to put your lips around the mouthpiece. The canister is depressed, the mist is suspended in the chamber, and the individual then takes several breaths in and out to get all the medicine available into the lung. The spacer has a special valve so that when you breathe out you are not blowing the medicine out of the spacer.

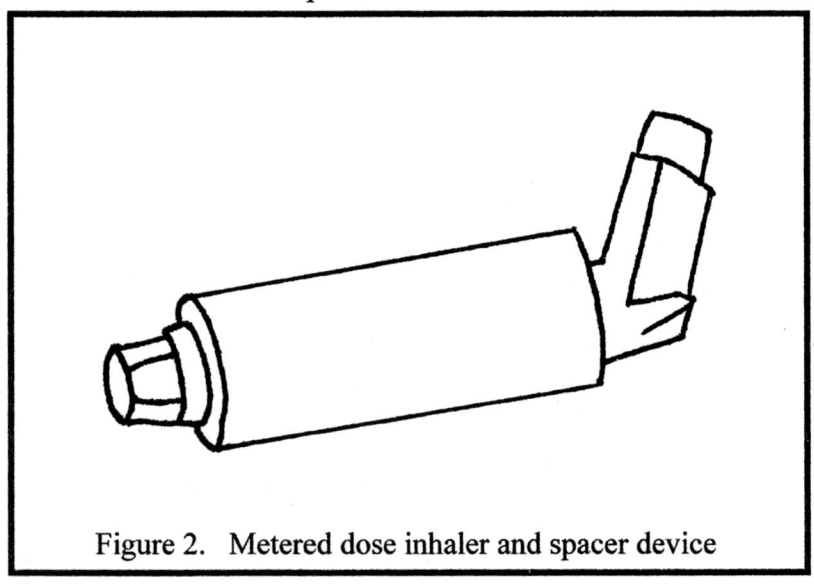

Figure 2. Metered dose inhaler and spacer device

Spacers are always recommended when using a steroid metered dose inhaler. This helps to deliver the optimal dose of medicine while reducing side effects. Spacers also work well with young children who are unable to use their rescue medication with the first technique described. Additionally, some spacers come with a soft plastic mask instead of a mouthpiece. This is very helpful for use with infants and toddlers. One steroid metered dose inhaler, Azmacort®, comes with a spacer already attached. However, it does not come with a facemask. Aerochamber®, is a commonly used spacer that comes with different size masks or a simple mouthpiece. You can use one spacer for all your metered dose inhalers.

ASSESSING ASTHMA SEVERITY: THE PEAK FLOW METER

Asthma symptoms are subjective and vary from person to person. The severity of asthma as expressed by someone's words may not fully define how short of breath they are. Some may complain of a tight cough, chest congestion, chest tightness, inability to take a deep breath, or chest pain. Obviously, these phrases can mean many things to many people. Children may have even more difficulty expressing how they feel because of a limited vocabulary or shyness. Other asthmatic individuals, suffering from chronic shortness of breath may feel only slightly worse, yet, have very little reserve left before their condition becomes critical. This makes the need for objective measurement of airflow a necessity.

The peak flow meter is a simple, inexpensive device used for the objective assessment of airflow out of the lung. There are several models of peak flow meters available, but, the design and use are much the same. Each meter consists of a long tube with a mouthpiece at one end, a small hole at the other end, and a moveable gauge between the two. (See Figure 3.)

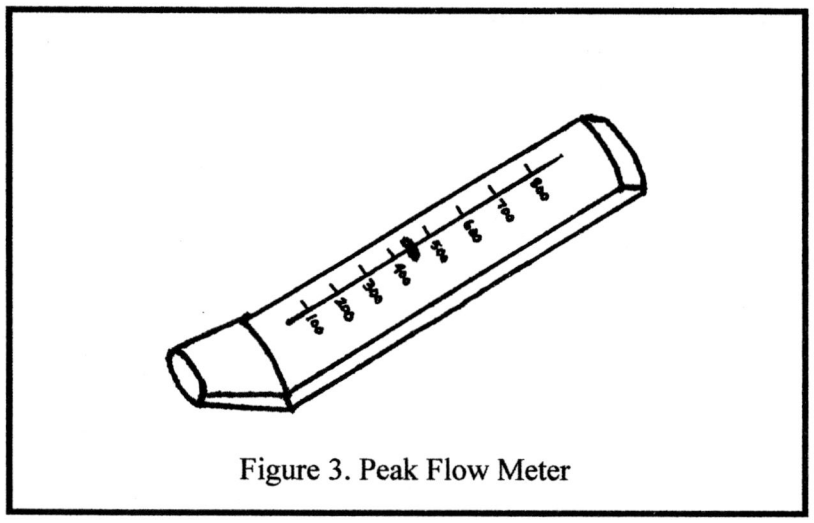

Figure 3. Peak Flow Meter

The peak flow meter measures the amount of air that can be exhaled from the lung over a period of time. While it may sound complex, in reality, it's just blowing hard through the tube. The idea is to get as much air out as possible in the shortest period of time. This effectively tells us how open or closed the bronchial airway is compared to when you feel well. The gauge on the meter moves along a numbered scale to indicate how much air was blown out. Just put your lips around the mouthpiece, take as deep a breath as possible and then blow as hard and as fast as you can. It is advised that you do this three times and take the best value as a current indication of your asthma severity. Be sure not to block the exit hole at the end of the meter while doing the procedure as it will give you a falsely high reading.

Each peak flow meter should come with a chart that indicates what the normal peak flow measurement should be based on age, height and sex. There can be some variability from one person to the next, but, for any given age, height and sex, the normal range should be within ten percent above or below this expected peak flow rate when healthy and unaffected by asthma symptoms. In patients with asthma, we want to know their "personal best" peak flow rate. This is the highest peak flow rate they have ever had when feeling well. All other measurements are compared to this one. For children, this number may increase over time as they continue to grow. When you are seen by a physician for increased asthma symptoms they may hand you a peak flow meter different than your own. This may yield slightly different results than your own meter, but, may still be used to monitor your progress with treatment.

The peak flow rate gives a more objective measure of bronchial airway narrowing. As the peak flow decreases, we can follow an individualized "asthma action plan" that will guide the asthmatic patient through a proper treatment regimen. This is especially helpful with children that are having trouble breathing. Generally, children age 4-5 can be taught to use a peak flow meter. They are more likely to use it correctly when they are asymptomatic. Children that do not feel well will often not attempt to use the peak flow meter. This can be a clue to increasing problems with asthma. Meters come in two sizes, one for adolescents and adults and one for children. Children using the adult meter are likely to have less reliable results. Keeping a record of daily peak flows is helpful in noting early decreases in airflow. This careful monitoring allows for early intervention.

Every asthmatic should have a peak flow meter and keep records on a regular basis. Anyone with a peak flow less than 50% of their personal best is advised to seek immediate medical attention. They may continue to take rescue medication while en route to see the doctor. Individuals with a peak flow rate between 50-80% of their personal best can use their rescue medication and recheck their peak flow rate after 10-15 minutes. If they are feeling worse, despite therapy, they should seek medical attention. If they are feeling better, they should continue their medications as prescribed and recheck their peak flow to make sure there is no further deterioration. Improvement following medication is indicated by a 10-20% increase in the peak flow.

Children that are unable to effectively use the peak flow meter on a regular basis should be evaluated by a physician for any signs of trouble breathing. This includes: rapid breathing; persistent cough; wheezing; mouth breathing with neck extended and head pushed forward; bluish discoloration to lips or fingers; inability to talk; lethargy; and retractions of the chest wall, where the ribs become prominent during respiration and the skin between the ribs gets "sucked in" with each breath.

COMMONLY ASKED QUESTIONS

Q: Who is qualified to evaluate and treat asthma? Should I see a specialist?

A: Many different medical specialties are qualified to evaluate and treat asthma. Some physicians may be more proficient than others based on knowledge and experience. Family physicians, pediatricians, allergists, internists, pulmonologists (lung specialist), and emergency room physicians are generally qualified to treat asthma. Many office-based physicians will be comfortable treating both acute asthma symptoms as well as managing routine asthma care. Other physicians may prefer to have you go to the local hospital emergency department for treatment of an acute asthma attack. Ask your doctor if they are comfortable managing both the acute and chronic care of your asthma. Ask if they think there is any value in seeing a specialist.

Q: Is allergy testing necessary? Do allergy shots help asthma?

A: Many patients with asthma can be and are successfully treated without having allergy testing. This is something that should be recommended on an individualized basis when suggested by the patient's history and current symptoms. For many individuals, taking the required steps in environmental changes mentioned previously is often enough to help decrease symptoms when used in addition to proper medication. It is important to remember that allergy testing, like all medical tests, have false positive and false negative results. The results may not be consistent with your experience. For example, you may test negative for allergy to cats, but, every time you're near a cat you're wheezing for several hours. Testing can help but it is not perfect by any means.

Allergy shots where small amounts of an allergic substance are injected through the skin, may have more value in preventing symptoms such as allergic rhinitis (itchy, watery nose) or the reaction from the venom of an insect sting. There is very little conclusive evidence that allergy shots will have a significant impact on asthma symptoms. This could be for a variety of reasons. It may be related to the fact that unidentified triggers remain and, therefore, are not included in the treatment regimen. It may be because the inflammatory process in the bronchial airway has progressed beyond where the shots can prevent it. Notably, if allergy shots were more beneficial for asthma, then, in all likelihood it would become the standard of care instead of inhaled steroids. Finally, it is important to remember that allergy shots are not without side effects. A severe anaphylactic reaction can occur with these injections. Individuals with moderate to severe asthma are advised not to receive allergy injections because of this risk. Remember that patients with chronic shortness of breath have less reserve when they become more short of breath. This type of reaction could have deadly consequences.

Q: I have recently been diagnosed with asthma. Will I have this problem the rest of my life?

A: This is a difficult question to answer. Asthma can be temporary, such as, Reactive Airways Dysfunction Syndrome. This will resolve with appropriate treatment in a few months if there is not repeated exposure. Other individuals can have a progressive course that does not improve despite multiple therapeutic interventions. The key to improving asthma is to identify as many triggers as possible, and avoid them. This, along with adequate medical therapy, may result in resolution of inflammation and improvement of symptoms. Some individuals will have a spontaneous recovery from asthma for unknown reasons. There is currently no way to know who will get better over time.

Q: My asthma symptoms do not occur every day. Do I need to take medication every day?

A: Current recommendations from the National Asthma Education and Prevention Program recommend daily anti-inflammatory prevention for anyone needing rescue medication more than twice weekly. This can be an inhaled steroid, a leukotriene inhibitor/blocker, cromolyn or nedocromil. If asthma is frequent, then treatment should be initiated with an inhaled steroid. If your asthma symptoms occur only with exercise, and you use a bronchodilator only for this purpose, then you do not necessarily need to use an anti-inflammatory medication.

Q: My daughter has asthma. Should I restrict her participation in sports like soccer or swimming? What about physical education classes at school?

A: This is a question best answered by your daughter's physician following a thorough exam. Asthma, in and of itself, should not be a reason to avoid athletic activity. Active participation requires that asthma be under good control. If asthma is worsened by exercise, then inhalation of a bronchodilator is recommended 15-20 minutes prior to starting exercise. Advise all coaches and physical education teachers of your child's condition. Send a letter and follow up with a phone call or a conversation at practice. Send a copy to the school nurse and principal as well. When asthma symptoms worsen, such as with a cold, your child should be excused from gym and athletic activities.

Q: My doctor recommends that I receive influenza (flu) vaccine every year. Is this really necessary?

A: Influenza virus is the cause of the flu. Specifically, the flu is an illness that includes fever, severe body aches, headache, runny and/or stuffy nose, sore throat and a dry to mildly productive cough. Vomiting sometimes occurs from the high fever and headaches. Diarrhea is uncommon. The virus infects the tissues lining the nose, throat and lungs. It is well known to cause worsening of asthma symptoms.

Vaccination currently involves an injection given annually in late autumn. Immunity develops in four to six weeks. Not everyone receiving the vaccine develops immunity for reasons that are unclear. The vaccine must be administered every year because the virus changes every year. A vaccine administered by nasal spray is currently under development and may be available in the fall of 2001. If you choose not to vaccinate, see your doctor as soon as symptoms develop. There are medications available that may shorten both the time and the severity of this illness. Consult with your physician.

Q: I'm on a high dose of prednisone because my asthma has been much worse lately. Can I still receive the influenza vaccine at this time?

A: There are published medical studies that show an individual can develop the appropriate immune response to vaccine while using steroid medication. Additionally, vaccination does not appear to make asthma worse assuming the individual is not allergic to any of the components of the vaccine, like eggs.

Q: My asthma becomes much worse whenever I have a cold. Can anything be done to prevent this?

A: This is a very common problem. Colds are caused by viruses and are transmitted from person to person, by close contact such as a sneeze in the face, drinking from the same cup, a handshake, handling the same object as someone with a cold, like a stair rail, a door handle or money. When we touch our hand to our nose or mouth, the virus infects us. Frequent hand washing is helpful to decrease the frequency of colds. This can be especially helpful at daycare, preschool and schools. If your asthma worsens with a cold, then call your doctor to discuss it. Many physicians will prescribe a short course of prednisone that may prevent worsening of asthma symptoms. This can be done for both adults and children.

Q: How often can I use rescue medication when I am short of breath?

A: The recommended dosing interval for most medications is 2 puffs every 4-6 hours. It is important to remember that these medications have an excellent safety profile and more frequent use is unlikely to cause a problem other than shakiness or rapid heart beat. More importantly, if you are in need of medication more often than recommended, then you need to ask why. If you improve after a few extra puffs, maybe that's fine. However, if you keep reaching for that inhaler every few minutes, then you need a more thorough evaluation by a qualified physician.

Q: Should I get a small volume nebulizer?

A: This device is best utilized by those individuals requiring high doses of rescue medication or those that cannot effectively use a metered dose inhaler with a spacer device. Consult with your physician.

Q: My asthma is always worse at night. I'm always coughing and waking up short of breath. What can I do?

A: Nocturnal asthma is a frequent problem for many people with asthma. The most important first step is avoidance of triggers and proper treatment of airway inflammation. Twice weekly changes of bed linen and sleepwear may be important in keeping the mite population at a minimum. Wash bed linens and sleepwear in hot water (140°F). If you suffer from acid reflux, take your medicine as prescribed and avoid eating or drinking alcohol for at least three hours before bedtime. Finally, ask your doctor about salmeterol (Serevent®). This is a long acting bronchodilator that should be taken about one hour prior to sleep. It works for up to twelve hours and may prevent airway narrowing during sleep. Check your morning peak flow against your personal best to help guide your therapy.

Q: After giving my child rescue medication for an acute attack of asthma, she stopped wheezing. Can I assume she is getting better?

A: **NO!** Don't be fooled. The absence of wheezing can be an ominous sign. Wheezing is a high pitched sound created by the movement of air through a narrowed airway. It has been estimated that wheezing can be heard with a stethoscope when

Why Do I Wheeze?

the airway is 70% of normal size. If you hear wheezing while standing next to someone, then the airway is probably more compromised. Additionally, not all asthmatics wheeze. Eventually, when asthma is severe, the airway is so narrow that little air passes through and wheezing becomes less apparent or even absent. Call 911 or any available emergency service as immediate intervention is critical. If wheezing goes away, peak flows go up and the asthmatic can speak freely and without hesitation, then you can be assured they are better.

Q: My child was treated with a nebulizer in the emergency department. Initially, he could barely talk. After the first treatment he could talk easier, but, I could hear him wheezing and that wasn't there before the treatment. Was he having an allergic reaction to the medicine?

A: No. It sounds like he was very short of breath. Once the medicine started to work, he could move enough air in and out of the lung to make the noise. This goes back to the last question. Remember, wheezing represents air movement, but, this time it means the patient is improving. With continued treatments, most of the wheezing should go away.

Q: Can too much rescue medication make asthma worse?

A: There is no good scientific evidence to suggest that too much rescue medication will worsen asthma. The safety of albuterol is evidenced by years of use throughout the world.. Emergency departments routinely give more than 10 milligrams of albuterol through nebulizers to the sickest asthmatic patients. This is more than fifty times the amount of albuterol in 2 puffs from a metered dose inhaler. A few years ago there were news reports of increasing asthma symptoms associated with more frequent use of metered dose inhalers. However, it is more likely that these individuals with increased shortness of breath had increased bronchial airway inflammation and were not responding to rescue medication in relatively small doses.

Q: Should my child have rescue medication available at school?

A: YES! The school nurse should have an inhaler handy for your child. Inform your child's teachers and have them tell your child it is all right if they need to leave class for medication. An extra peak flow meter at the nurse's office may also be helpful. Be sure the nurse is aware of your child's personal best peak flow rate. Keep the number current as your child grows.

Q: Recently, I had a cold, cough and fever. My asthma became much worse. Would an antibiotic help?

A: There are multiple infectious agents that may worsen asthma. Most of these agents are viruses. With the exception of the flu virus, there is no current treatment to directly affect cold viruses. Most antibiotics are active against bacteria that may complicate viral illnesses. A good example is sinusitis. With a cold virus, there is swelling, congestion and fluid accumulation in the nose and sinuses. Bacteria, already present in the nose and sinuses may start to grow and multiply in the sinuses. This results in inflammation of the sinuses. There is increased swelling and increased pain as the body's immune system fights the infection. This is a case where antibiotics are needed. Additionally, in the asthmatic patient, steroids may be important as sinusitis can cause a flare up of asthma. Finally, any infection of the lung can cause worsening of asthma. Bronchitis, an acute bronchial infection is usually viral. If it persists beyond a couple of weeks an antibiotic trial may be helpful.

It is important to remember that antibiotics are not routinely indicated for colds or bronchitis. Antibiotics should be used selectively to prevent the development of resistance and to avoid unnecessary side effects.

Q: I'm pregnant. Can I continue my asthma medication?

A: Yes. Asthma medication, specifically, inhaled steroids and rescue medication have been used for years in pregnancy with no documented ill effects to mother or child. Poorly controlled asthma may be detrimental to the fetus if oxygen supply is reduced with severe symptoms. Intermittent use of high dose steroids can be helpful for severe episodes of asthma without significant harm to the fetus. High dose steroids throughout the pregnancy is probably not safe. If you are trying to get pregnant, make sure your asthma is under control and follow up with your physician regularly.

Q: Can I nurse my infant while using asthma medication? Will it affect the baby?

A: There are no medical studies that can help predict how much medicine will be concentrated in breast milk. High dose oral steroids are probably going to have some effect on infants such as slowing the growth rate. However, it is unlikely that inhaled steroids will cause any significant problem as they are rapidly metabolized by the body. Breast feeding has many important attributes for infants that far outweigh the risk from inhaled steroids. Rescue medication is unlikely to cause any problems.

Q: I have heard many stories about the side effects of steroids. Are they safe to use? Do they affect my child's growth?

A: Inhaled steroids are safe. They have been used for years in both children and adults. Some studies have suggested that growth rates slow in children while other studies have not demonstrated this effect. The rate of growth may be decreased by 1-2 centimeters per year. Overall, the final height is unaffected. However, there are no good studies to tell how much growth is affected in children with severe asthma that do not receive appropriate treatment.

Inhaled steroids have been suspected as a potential cause of cataracts, but, this remains to be proven conclusively. Inhaled steroids can cause yeast infections in the mouth. Treatment with anti-fungal antibiotics is usually successful. Using a spacer with a steroid inhaler and rinsing the mouth after use is preventive.

Oral steroids have proven very effective and safe for short periods of time (less than 7-10 days). However, recurrent use can weaken muscles and bone, cause cataracts, weight gain, water retention and make control of diabetes more difficult. It can also suppress the body's ability to respond to stress, such as surgery or infection. This can lead to other complications such as very low blood pressure. These side effects are uncommon with inhaled steroids.

Q: Are there useful medications available for asthma that can be bought without a prescription?

A: There are tablets and inhalers available over-the-counter for asthma. These medications can have some bronchodilating effect. The available inhalers offer medication that has a short duration of action, and, as such, may require very frequent use to maintain adequate breathing. These medications are much less effective than prescription rescue medication. Additionally, they offer no anti-inflammatory effect. Avoid these medications. See your doctor for appropriate treatment.

Q: I feel my heart racing in my chest after using rescue medication. Is this normal? Is it safe?

A: This is a side effect of the medication. While it is not common it can occur and usually resolves rapidly. It is more common in patients that have had multiple nebulizer treatments or an injection of adrenaline or terbutaline. If your heart is healthy this is generally not a problem. Individuals with heart disease or angina may have worsening of their heart pains if their heart starts racing. Additionally, wheezing can be a sign of congestive heart failure, and, you don't want to treat that like asthma. Tell your doctor if you have a history of heart disease.

Q: Unfortunately, I found out a while ago that I am allergic to cats. I gave away my cat but I'm still having trouble breathing. How come?

A: Despite adequate cleaning, cat dander can be found 6 months after the cat has departed. Continued cleaning will be necessary along with appropriate anti-inflammatory medication. Remember, additional triggers may be present yet unidentified.

Q: I always sneeze and wheeze a few hours after I visit my sister's house. Is this allergy related?

A: It may be. You're probably not allergic to your sister though. It may represent allergy to something in the house such as animal dander, plant material, smoke or some other substance. It is not unusual for allergic reactions to be delayed by several hours following exposure to triggering agents. Thus, an allergic reaction can be initiated by contact at one location but not become symptomatic until you are somewhere else. This is an important point to consider when trying to identify triggering agents that can worsen asthma symptoms.

Q: My doctor says that my asthma is caused from acid backing up from my stomach into my esophagus. I didn't have any symptoms, but, my doctor ordered a special x-ray test and found the problem. I'm using medication to decrease acid production. How soon can I expect to feel an improvement in my asthma?

A: If acid reflux is the only cause of your asthma, then improvement should occur over a 2-6 month period. This presumes continued treatment with medication to decrease acid secretion from the stomach as well as continued anti-inflammatory therapy. Some individuals will have persistent reflux despite multiple medical therapies. Some of these individuals will benefit from anti-reflux surgery.

It is important to note that reflux can occur with or without symptoms. It is often overlooked as a cause of asthma for this reason. If you have persistent asthma without an identifiable cause, ask your doctor about doing tests for reflux. Finally, it should be noted that asthma does not occur in the majority of people with reflux.

Q: My son is 18 months old and was recently diagnosed with an "RSV" infection. He had a high fever, runny nose, cough and wheezing. Does he have asthma?

A: Respiratory Syncytial Virus, or RSV, is an infection of the bronchial airway. As an infectious process, it causes inflammation that can lead to shortness of breath and wheezing. Bronchospasm may also occur. There are studies that suggest RSV may be a trigger that promotes a tendency toward asthma. However, it would not be accurate to diagnose someone with asthma just because they tested positive for RSV and have shortness of breath and wheezing.

Q: Is there any treatment for RSV?

A: Most children that get RSV do not wheeze. Simple treatment with acetaminophen (Tylenol®) for fever and plenty of fluids to prevent dehydration is all that is needed. Those children with cough and wheezing are often treated with bronchodilators. The response to bronchodilators varies from child to child. Steroids have not been proven effective at reducing the severity of this illness. Ribavirin®, is an RSV specific medication that is given to hospitalized children with severe infection. This drug slows the amount of virus produced within the airway. It is not an anti-inflammatory medication nor is it a bronchodilator.

Q: How do you test for RSV?

A: RSV is found in nasal secretions. Typically, a sample of nasal fluid must be obtained from the back of the nose. A cotton tipped applicator may be inserted to collect the sample or a salt water solution is squirted into the back of the nose and then sucked out again. The sample is then tested in a laboratory. The accuracy of this test is dependent on many factors, but, in general is very reliable.

Q: My doctor prescribed an inhaled steroid because I have persistent symptoms. Should I take it every day or just when I need it?

A: Inhaled steroids should be used every day. Inhaled steroids do not work immediately. They work over a prolonged period of time to decrease activity in the white blood cells that cause inflammation. Don't stop your inhaled steroid just because you feel better. Consult with your physician prior to discontinuing any medication.

Q: I know the doctor says I need to use my inhaled steroid everyday, however, I'm concerned about side effects. Are there other medications available with fewer side effects?

A: There are other medications that may be helpful. However, inhaled steroids are probably the best treatment initially for anyone with persistent asthma. Leukotriene inhibitors/blockers, cromolyn or nedocromil may be helpful. Some individuals will be able to maintain stable asthma with these other medications but most will require inhaled steroids.

Q: We have made three trips to the emergency room with our daughter in the past six months. Her asthma seems to be getting worse each time. What can we do?

A: This is a complicated question with many answers. First, go throughout the living space to look for potential triggers and remove them. Next, look at other possible sources. Does your child spend a lot of time at daycare or at another person's house after school? Is there a trigger at school? Are symptoms better by Monday morning? Does her asthma only get worse with cold symptoms? Is she taking her medicine correctly? Does the dose of her medication need to be increased? Check with your doctor and ask if she should see a specialist.

Q: My asthma is well controlled except just prior to and during my menstrual period. Is this common? What can be done?

A: The association between increased asthma symptoms and menstrual flow is well documented. It does not appear to be common. Some studies have suggested that birth control pills are beneficial. The cause is unknown but thought to be related to fluctuations in hormone levels.

Q: I always get headaches, swelling in my legs and indigestion when I use prednisone tablets. Can I just increase the amount of inhaled steroid when my asthma worsens instead of using prednisone? Is there an alternative to prednisone?

A: It is possible to increase the dose of inhaled steroid when asthma worsens. However, if you are not breathing well, the amount of medicine that is actually deposited in the bronchial airway may not be as much as needed. Your symptoms may worsen more because of this. Additionally, you may suffer more local side effects from the increased dose, such as a fungal infection of the mouth. There are several other oral steroids available. Explain your side effects to your physician and ask to try a different oral steroid.

Q: I recently read that individuals using steroid medication are more prone to colds, tonsillitis and pneumonia. Is this true?

A: No. The above illnesses are caused by infectious viruses and bacteria. While steroids do slow the immune system down, it does not affect your chances of getting one these diseases. One exception is yeast infection. Individuals using inhaled steroids are more prone to a yeast infection of the mouth. The frequency of this infection can be greatly reduced by using a spacer device when inhaling the medicine and rinsing the mouth after each use.

Q: Asthma is much more common today. Why?

A: There are many theories about the increase in asthma over the past ten to twenty years. The increase in childhood asthma may be related to increased time in a daycare setting. Children in daycare have twice the number of colds as children that stay at home. They also have more frequent ear infections. Asthma symptoms may be provoked by frequent inflammation of the nose and sinuses associated with a cold. With less time to recover between illnesses, the inflammatory process becomes chronic and may trigger asthma symptoms.

Lifestyle changes may also play a role in asthma development. Our bed linens are colored and washed in cold water, not hot. This may result in a higher mite population. The content of our diet may increase the risk of asthma. "Fast food" is a regular meal several times a week for many children as well as adults. As a population, we are overweight, putting us at risk for gastroesophageal reflux. The air quality in our cities and within the home may be another trigger. Newer homes are often built so well that fresh air does not enter except when a door or window is opened. Allergens may be constantly recycled through the air if not filtered out somehow. Additionally, our technology rich industries require many chemicals to produce various products. These chemicals may cause occupational asthma. This is a brief list of possibilities with many more yet to be discovered.

Q: Do I need to use a spacer for all my asthma medication?

A: No. The spacer is recommended for use with inhaled steroids to reduce side effects. It is also recommended that small children use this with their rescue medication to enhance delivery to the airway. When used appropriately, rescue medication can be used without a spacer. If you hold the inhaler one to two inches from your lips as you depress it, then your open mouth effectively becomes a spacer.

Q: The emergency room doctor gave our son both albuterol and ipratropium in a nebulizer treatment. Is it safe to mix these drugs? Do two drugs work better than one?

A: Ipratropium and Albuterol have been mixed together in nebulizer treatments for years. They are very safe to give together. They work to relieve bronchospasm by two different mechanisms. However, there is uncertainty whether ipratropium provides any additional benefit to albuterol. Most patients will get better with albuterol alone in the same amount of time as those that get both medications.

Q: My asthma is a constant battle. Despite years of treatment and attempts to control my environmental triggers, I am short of breath every day. My doctor says I am resistant to the beneficial effects of steroids, including high dose oral steroids. What can be done?

A: You are not alone. Many asthmatics have been labeled steroid resistant. More recent medical research indicates that these individuals require much higher doses of steroid medication in order to get the same response. Additionally, they require a longer treatment period, slowly decreasing their daily dose over a prolonged time. Increased side effects can be expected. Inhaled steroids should be continued throughout the course of treatment as well as regular visits to your physician.
    There are other medications being used to treat the inflammation of asthma. Methotrexate is a medicine used for treating cancer that has been found helpful in some asthmatic patients. It should be prescribed only by physicians familiar with its use and potential side effects.
    The future for asthma treatment is hopeful with many new medications being studied in research centers.

Q: My doctor has recommended sinus surgery after years of chronic sinusitis. Will this help my asthma as well as my sinusitis?

A: Unfortunately, there is no good evidence to suggest that sinus surgery will improve asthma symptoms. This does not mean you should not have the surgery. While the surgery may not help to improve your asthma symptoms, perhaps it will prevent your asthma from progressing to a more severe form.

Q: What is the purpose of an Asthma Action Plan?

A: The Asthma Action Plan is a guide for treatment depending on symptoms and peak flow measurements. The plan is based on your personal best peak flow rate given your sex, height and age. Specific instructions for medication use are given as well as appropriate actions to take if asthma does not improve with symptoms. A copy of the North Shore Asthma Clinic "Asthma Action Plan" is included with your book.

Q: The emergency room doctor insisted on giving steroids to my wife through an intravenous (IV) catheter. Is this better than taking the steroid by mouth?

A: There is no additional anti-inflammatory effect to be gained by giving steroids through the IV. If the patient has been vomiting, then this becomes a rational choice. Additionally, in patients with severe asthma, an IV may be helpful for giving other medications, such as the bronchodilator terbutaline. Also, if breathing is severely restricted, the doctor may not want the patient to swallow because it may briefly interfere with breathing or potentially cause a choking episode with further deterioration of the patients condition.

Why Do I Wheeze?

Q: Recently, I was treated at an urgent care center for asthma. I had a bad cold and my asthma worsened. I explained to the doctor that I was ten weeks along in my first pregnancy. I received multiple breathing treatments and felt better, however, the doctor would not prescribe any steroid medication because of the pregnancy. The next night my symptoms became much worse. Should I have received a steroid medication?

A: YES! This omission is the most likely reason for your relapse. A short course of steroid treatment should have no long term impact on the growing fetus. Severe asthma can result in decreased oxygen in the blood stream and this can be harmful to mother and fetus. If this happens to you, call your personal physician and explain what happened. You need the appropriate treatment.

Q: I recently saw an asthma specialist. I have severe persistent asthma and have been doing poorly with many different treatments. The doctor has recommended a treatment with an intravenous medication called gamma globulin. Is this new? Is it safe?

A: Gamma globulin has been used safely for many years. It is made up of antibodies from the serum of many people. The serum is the liquid part of the blood without the red and white blood cells. Antibodies help to fight infection and also help to neutralize substances that may be causing an illness. There is research showing a positive effect of gamma globulin in asthmatic patients. This treatment is relatively expensive and usually reserved for only the sickest patients that have failed other forms of therapy.

Q: Is any one inhaled steroid better than another?

A: All of the currently approved inhaled steroids are effective. Individual patients may feel an improved response with one versus another. Likewise, side effects may differ slightly from person to person. If you feel your medicine is not helping you or it doesn't agree with you for some other reason, tell your doctor, there are alternatives to try.

Q: Are there any herbal remedies that improve asthma?

A: There is a considerable amount of literature about the benefit of herbal remedies. Most reports come from China and Japan as they have longed utilized herbal remedies for medicinal purposes. It is difficult to assess the value of any one herbal product because they are rarely, if ever, a solitary substance. Rather, most of these medications are made up of numerous substances in varying amount. This is in no way meant to deny value to these products. It only points out that consistent benefit may not always be obtainable due to variation in the concentration of various chemicals. How often and how much of any one herbal medicine is needed for an effect is often unknown. Additionally, it is reported that these remedies can be contaminated by other leaf extracts or herbs that could be detrimental to your condition. They could cause an allergic reaction and/or stimulate more inflammation within the airway. Finally, it should be remembered that even natural substances used to treat illness can have side effects as well as interact negatively with your other medications. Before you consider an herbal or natural remedy for asthma, read as much about it as possible. Tell your doctor you want to try something different and why.

Q: Why don't the drug companies study herbs to produce the active ingredient?

A: Money. It costs up to $500 million to bring a drug to market from discovery through final FDA approval. Medicines derived from plant material are not necessarily covered by patent rights. Once developed, a large pharmaceutical company could lose all potential costs to develop as well as profits to a generic drug maker. By the way, cromolyn comes from a plant.

Q: My doctor wants to add a leukotriene blocker to my list of medicines. I already use a steroid inhaler and Serevent® every day. Is this safe? Will I be able to stop my other medications?

A: A leukotriene blocker may provide additional benefit to your current treatment regimen. It is safe to administer with your inhaled medications. Some individuals have been successfully weaned off inhaled steroids after starting a leukotriene blocker. Still, others may receive no additional benefit. Do not suddenly stop using your inhaled steroid when starting this medication. A gradual withdrawal, perhaps one less puff per day, every five or six days, while closely monitoring peak flow changes, is required. Consult with your physician if your condition worsens or if you think you are having side effects from the medication.

Q: I inhale my steroid medication from a device that delivers a powder, not a spray. Do I need a spacer?

A: No. The medication within this device is designed to be inhaled directly without a spacer. You should rinse your mouth with water after each use to prevent a possible yeast infection in the mouth.

Q: I have had a chronic sinus infection for months. I am currently completing my third course of antibiotics in the past six weeks. My nose continues to drain a thick discharge and I don't feel there has been any improvement. What could be wrong?

A: There are a number of possibilities. First, an infection of this duration should be cultured to identify the causative bacteria and tested to find out which antibiotic is most appropriate. If no bacteria are identified, it may indicate another cause such as allergy, chronic inflammation from an infection that is now cleared, or, more rarely, a foreign body in the nose. Children with chronic drainage of pus from the nose have occasionally been found to have a bead or small pebble up their nose.

Initial treatment should include use of a topical decongestant spray for no more than three days. This should be followed by daily treatment with a steroid nasal spray. Antibiotic therapy should be based on culture results to avoid overuse and potential side effects. A thorough physical exam by an ear, nose and throat specialist, and in selected cases, a CT scan of the sinuses may be helpful in identifying a cause.

Q: I have allergic rhinitis during the fall hayfever season. I noticed that it was not as severe this past year while taking a leukotriene blocker. Is this related?

A: Yes. Many individuals have reported improvement in various allergy symptoms after starting these medications. Leukotrienes are secreted in the body in response to allergy as part of the inflammatory process. However, not all individuals will benefit from this treatment.

Why Do I Wheeze?

Q: Recently, my husband was taken to the emergency room for a severe asthma attack. He was so short of breath he couldn't talk. The emergency room physician treated him with magnesium intravenously, helium and oxygen through a mask over his face as well as multiple injections of adrenaline. It took a while but he did improve to the point where he could talk again. Are all these medications necessary?

A: When faced with such a difficult situation it is not unusual to try every possible therapy. Medical research has suggested but not proven that there may be some benefit to helium inhalation when administered with oxygen. It appears to flow through the narrowed airways more smoothly than pure oxygen. Magnesium is well known for its ability to relax smooth muscles in the uterus for preterm labor and is thought to be helpful as a bronchodilator. However, it has yet to be proven to be any more beneficial than just using the usual bronchodilating medication.

Q: My daughter uses an inhaled steroid daily. Without it, her asthma worsens quickly. I'm very concerned about it affecting her growth. Is there anything I can do?

A: Medical research suggests that growth may be slowed by one-two centimeters per year while using inhaled steroids. There are other studies that fail to show any difference. Final height is unaffected. Further, the studies are inconclusive about whether persistent severe asthma affects growth. There is some research to support the use of inhaled steroids in the daytime to prevent any delay in growth. Growth generally takes place during sleep. It has been suggested that morning administration of the daily dose of inhaled steroid may prevent growth delay. However, some individuals may have worsening symptoms related to once daily dosing. Consult your physician before changing your medication routine.

Q: My child complains of chest pain when running at school. She appears out of breath and frequently stops the prescribed activity due to this discomfort. This has not been a problem when playing vigorously at home and testing at the doctor's office did not show any problems. What could be wrong?

A: There are several possibilities. This could be exercise induced asthma. This could be related to some other issues at school itself. It is important to test for asthma in the actual school setting. There could be a triggering agent in the school that causes some minor bronchospasm and this is worsened by exercise. One study revealed a student reacting to the cat dander on the clothes of a fellow student. Additionally, many school buildings are old, dusty and may be a significant source of mold or other allergens. Do peak flows before going to school on Monday morning, then before, during and after gym class. If peak flows fall from the morning reading, consult with your physician about appropriate treatment. Finally, talk with school administrators about potential triggers in the school environment.

Q: What changes in asthma therapy can we expect in the near future?

A: There are a large number of medications currently being tested for asthma. Most are directed at altering the process of inflammation. It is unlikely that any one drug will be a "magic bullet". Preventive treatment and environmental control will still be necessary. The metered dose inhaler will become less frequently used as powdered medication becomes more popular and easy to use. Most powder medications will not require the use of a spacer. Additionally, you can expect to see medications combined into one inhaler. For example, your daily anti-inflammatory medication will be combined with a broncho-dilator that has a prolonged duration of action.

Why Do I Wheeze?

Q: I received a prednisone prescription when I was discharged from the hospital emergency department. The instructions said to take six pills for two days, four pills for two days, two pills for two days then one pill for two days. Why?

A: This is called a steroid taper. Steroids have been prescribed in a similar fashion for years despite no scientific evidence to its effectiveness when compared with taking the same dose every day for five days. It was thought that a tapered dose would allow for the body's adrenal gland to resume normal steroid production and reduce potential steroid withdrawal side effects. This tapering dose may still be useful for individuals that are severely ill and require daily oral steroids as their adrenal glands may secrete very little cortisol. However, for asthma patients with an occasional flare up, a brief five day course of oral steroids without a taper is both safe and effective.

Q: I have a friend that states her asthma has never been better since she started an herbal remedy. What is in the herbs that is so helpful?

A: It is difficult to know the contents because there are no regulations requiring the manufacturer to list all of the ingredients. Many individuals get better from the placebo effect. They believe the medicine will work and so it does. This is true for many medicines given for many illnesses. It is possible that some ingredient could exert an anti-inflammatory effect. The real question is, will the next pill or the next bottle contain the same medication or the same amount per pill? No one can be sure. There is one known case where the manufacturer was adding prednisone to the remedy without including this on the label. Yes, people felt better! Buyer beware.

GLOSSARY

allergen: a substance capable of stimulating or binding to white blood cells resulting in a reaction in the body that may include swelling of affected areas, increased fluid secretion (such as watery eyes and nose), shortness of breath, wheezing or low blood pressure. Examples of allergens include pollen, bee venom, nuts, cats, latex.

alveoli: the air sacs at the end of the bronchial air passageway. this is the site where oxygen and carbon dioxide are exchanged to and from the blood, respectively.

asthma: a disease that results in narrowing of the bronchial air passageways as a result of inflammation and/or bronchospasm.

bronchus (bronchi): the air passageway(s) of the lung that carry air into and out of the lung.

bronchoconstriction: refers to narrowing of the air passageways due to inflammation, bronchospasm, or both. This results in decreased air flow through the lung and subsequent shortness of breath.

bronchodilation: refers to opening or enlarging the air passageway allowing more air to flow in and out of the lung.

bronchodilator: refers to medication that helps to open or enlarge the air passageways. Also called rescue medication. Helps to relieve bronchospasm and may enhance the ability to cough up secretions within the airway.

bronchospasm: refers to the contraction or squeezing of muscle around the bronchial airway causing it to narrow and resulting in shortness of breath

early (immediate) asthmatic response: shortness of breath that develops within seconds or minutes following contact with a triggering agent or allergen.

exercise induced asthma (EIA): asthma brought on by exercise, usually starting a few minutes after activity level has increased and persisting for several minutes thereafter; may resolve spontaneously in some individuals while others may need rescue medication.

gastroesophageal reflux (GERD): a process involving the backward flow of stomach acid and food into the esophagus. a commonly overlooked cause of asthma.

house-dust mite: a microscopic insect that eats dead skin from animals and people. a common cause of allergy and asthma.

inflammation: a protective response of the body to injury. typically involves swelling of affected areas with fluid, chemicals secreted by white blood cells, and the accumulation of white blood cells to prevent damage from foreign substances. this process is common in chronic asthma and becomes damaging instead of protective.

late phase asthmatic response: shortness of breath that develops hours or days after initial contact with a triggering agent.

metered dose inhaler: a device consisting of a canister containing medication and a holder with a mouthpiece that allows for the delivery of a specified amount of medication with each depression of the canister within its holder.

Nocturnal asthma: asthma that occurs during sleep. may result in frequent awakenings or persistent cough. Affected individuals may sleep through episode without realizing airflow is decreased.

small volume nebulizer: a device for delivery of liquid medication as an aerosol. Air or oxygen flows through a small hose into a medication holding chamber producing a fine mist which can be inhaled, delivering medication directly to the bronchial airway.

spacer device: a hollow chamber for use with a metered dose inhaler. This allows for suspension of medication within the device, resulting in improved delivery of medicine to the bronchial airway when inhaled.

spirometry: a group of breathing tests that quantify the amount of airflow through the lungs providing information on how well air flows in and out of the lung.

triggering agent: any substance capable of provoking an allergic reaction, bronchospasm or bronchial inflammation.

APPENDIX

BRONCHODILATORS

Albuterol: Proventil®, Ventolin®

Metaproterenol: Alupent®

Bitolterol: Tornalate®

Pirbuterol: Maxair®

Terbutaline: Brethaire®, Brethine®

Ipratropium: Atrovent®

Salmeterol: Serevent® (metered dose inhaler or powder)

Albuterol/Ipratropium: Combivent®

LEUKOTRIENE INHIBITORS/BLOCKERS

Zafirlukast: Accolate® (available for age 7 and above)

Montelukast: Singulair® (available for age 6 and above)

Zileuton: Zyflo®

INHALED STEROIDS

Beclomethasone: Beclovent®, Vanceril®

Triamcinolone: Azmacort®

Fluticasone: Flovent® (metered dose inhaler or powder)

Budesonide: Pulmicort® (powder)

Flunisolide: Aerobid®

THEOPHYLLINE

Marax®   Slo-Bid®   Theo-24®   Theo-Dur®

Uni-Dur®   Uniphyl®

NOTES

NOTES

NOTES

NOTES

NOTES

NOTES

NOTES

NOTES

To order additional copies of Why Do I Wheeze?, complete the information below or order directly from our web site at **www.whydoiwheeze.com**

Ship To: (please print)

Name _____

Address _____

City, State, Zip _____

Daytime Phone _____

____ copies of Why Do I Wheeze? @ $14.95 each $_____

Postage and handling @ $1.95 per book $_____

Total amount enclosed $_____

Method of Payment:
Check/Money order payable to: North Shore Asthma Clinic

VISA____   Mastercard____

Name on card _____

Card Number __ __ __ __ - __ __ __ __ - __ __ __ __ - __ __ __ __

Exp. Date_____   Cardholder Signature_____

Send order to: North Shore Asthma Clinic
                1950 Sheridan Rd Suite 202
                Highland Park, IL 60035

Please allow 10 business days for delivery.

To order additional copies of Why Do I Wheeze?, complete the information below or order directly from our web site at www.whydoiwheeze.com

Ship To: (please print)

Name _____

Address _____

City, State, Zip _____

Daytime Phone _____

_____ copies of Why Do I Wheeze? @ $14.95 each $_____

Postage and handling @ $1.95 per book $_____

Total amount enclosed $_____

Method of Payment:
Check/Money order payable to: North Shore Asthma Clinic

VISA_____   Mastercard_____

Name on card _____

Card Number __ __ __ __ - __ __ __ __ - __ __ __ __ - __ __ __ __

Exp. Date _____   Cardholder Signature _____

Send order to: North Shore Asthma Clinic
1950 Sheridan Rd Suite 202
Highland Park, IL 60035

Please allow 10 business days for delivery.

To order additional copies of Why Do I Wheeze?, complete the information below or order directly from our web site at www.whydoiwheeze.com

Ship To: (please print)

Name _____

Address _____

City, State, Zip _____

Daytime Phone _____

____ copies of Why Do I Wheeze? @ $14.95 each $_____

      Postage and handling @ $1.95 per book $_____

                    Total amount enclosed $_____

Method of Payment:
Check/Money order payable to: North Shore Asthma Clinic

VISA____   Mastercard____

Name on card _____

Card Number __ __ __ __ - __ __ __ __ - __ __ __ __ - __ __ __ __

Exp. Date _____   Cardholder Signature _____

Send order to: North Shore Asthma Clinic
               1950 Sheridan Rd Suite 202
               Highland Park, IL 60035

Please allow 10 business days for delivery.

To order additional copies of Why Do I Wheeze?, complete the information below or order directly from our web site at **www.whydoiwheeze.com**

Ship To: (please print)

Name _____

Address _____

City, State, Zip _____

Daytime Phone _____

____ copies of Why Do I Wheeze? @ $14.95 each $_____

    Postage and handling @ $1.95 per book $_____

               Total amount enclosed $_____

Method of Payment:
Check/Money order payable to: North Shore Asthma Clinic

VISA____   Mastercard____

Name on card _____

Card Number __ __ __ __ - __ __ __ __ - __ __ __ __ - __ __ __ __

Exp. Date_____   Cardholder Signature _____

Send order to: North Shore Asthma Clinic
                1950 Sheridan Rd Suite 202
                Highland Park, IL 60035

Please allow 10 business days for delivery.

To order additional copies of Why Do I Wheeze?, complete the information below or order directly from our web site at **www.whydoiwheeze.com**

Ship To: (please print)

Name _____

Address _____

City, State, Zip _____

Daytime Phone _____

____ copies of Why Do I Wheeze? @ $14.95 each $_____

    Postage and handling @ $1.95 per book $_____

        Total amount enclosed $_____

Method of Payment:
Check/Money order payable to: North Shore Asthma Clinic

VISA____   Mastercard____

Name on card _____

Card Number __ __ __ __ - __ __ __ __ - __ __ __ __ - __ __ __ __

Exp. Date_____   Cardholder Signature_____

Send order to: North Shore Asthma Clinic
               1950 Sheridan Rd Suite 202
               Highland Park, IL 60035

Please allow 10 business days for delivery.